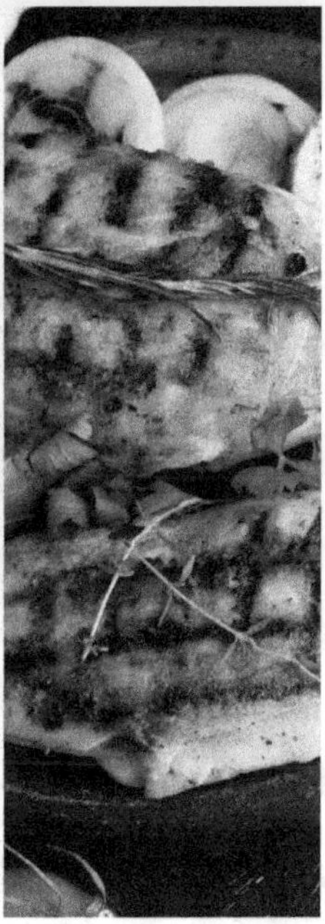

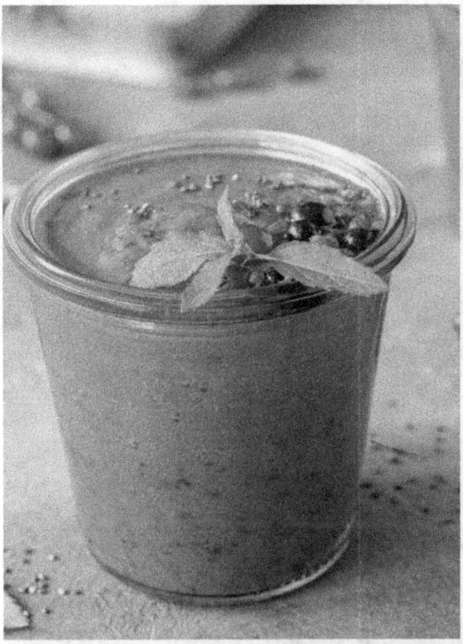

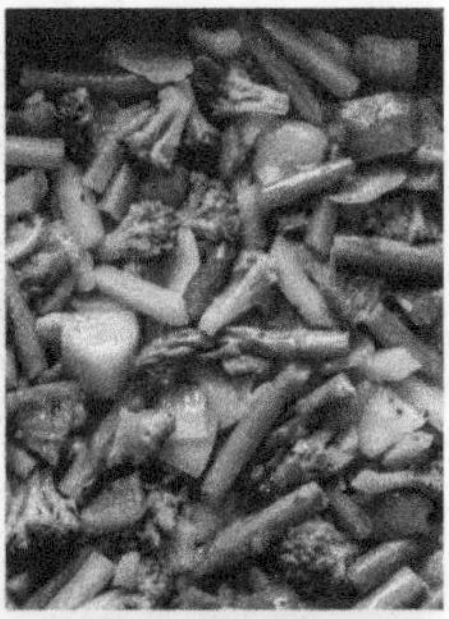

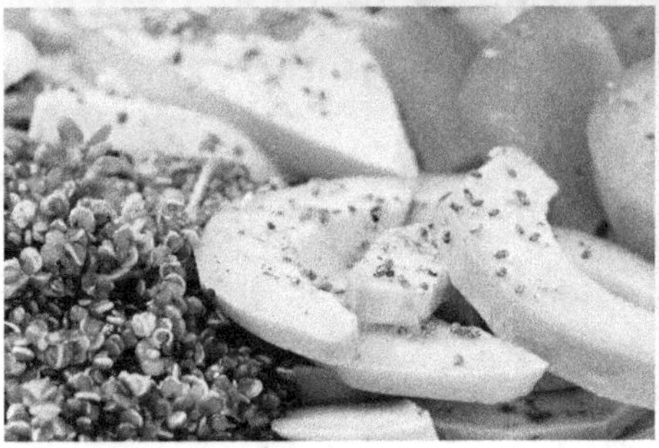

THE
HORMONAL
BALANCE
PLAN FOR
WOMEN

A Guide to Regain Your Well-being, Shedding Pounds, and Restoring Your Vitality

By

Dr. FAWN ROSE

Copyright (c) 2023 by Dr. FAWN ROSE

The greatest sources accessible at the time of writing served as the foundation for the material in this book. Regarding the correctness or completeness of the contents of this book, the author and the publisher make no claims or warranties, either express or implicit, and they explicitly disclaim any implied warranties of merchantability or suitability for a particular purpose. The publisher and author disclaim all liability for any loss or damage resulting from or related to the use of this book.

The sole goal of this book is to be informative. The publisher and author do not provide any professional, legal, or medical advice. Should you need such guidance, please contact a qualified expert.

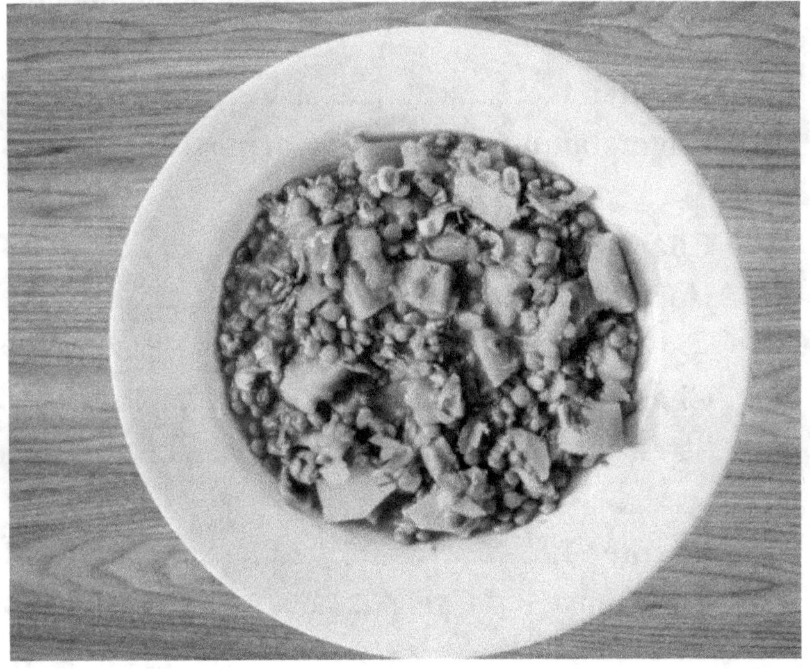

Table of contents

Introduction

Hormones are powerful chemical messengers that play a subtle but significant role in the complex and amazing fabric of human life. These inconspicuous molecules have an intricate role in regulating our general health and well-being by coordinating a complex symphony of physiological events. Women are among the many groups that benefit from the balanced interaction of hormones. Women's hormone balancing is an amazing and always-changing experience with many distinct chapters.

Titled "The Hormonal Balance Plan for Women," this extensive book takes us on a trip that goes beyond science and biology. It's an investigation of the complexities of female hormone systems, their significant influence on many facets of life, and the skill of maintaining a balanced, harmonious hormonal equilibrium. This journey isn't linear; rather, it's a vast tale that spans many life phases, with each chapter presenting its own set of obstacles and successes. This book chronicles the ever-present, ever-changing hormones and their profound effects on women's growth, development, emotional well-being, and general health. It covers the stages of life from the innocence of childhood to turbulent adolescence, the complexity of adulthood, the transformative middle age, and the graceful embrace of older years.

Our starting point is an understanding of women's hormones. We explore the complex systems and finely balanced hormones that characterize a woman's health, realizing that these unseen conductors affect not only the physical but also the emotional and psychological aspects of existence. Our next topic of study will be hormonal imbalances, which present a serious problem and have a dramatic effect on women's health in a variety of ways. Understanding and successfully resolving these issues requires an awareness of the telltale indications and symptoms of these imbalances.

Now let's talk about nutrition. We discover that the delicate hormonal balance may be supported by the foods we eat. All of the meals—breakfast, lunch, supper, and snacks—become instruments for promoting hormonal balance all day long. Our following chapter delves into the deep effects of stress on hormone balance and provides insight into strategies that protect the sacredness of hormonal health.

We examine the many stages of the menstrual cycle and how hormone fluctuations affect mood and food desires. Hormone optimization enables us to identify techniques for keeping a healthy weight in the fight against the bulge.

The focus of our study then turns to hormones and their impact on reproductive health and fertility. Improving hormonal balance is essential for improving reproductive health. We provide the resources that enable women to travel toward increased fertility.

The transforming path of aging gracefully is introduced in Chapter 8. Hormonal changes that occur throughout perimenopause and menopause are discussed, and methods for symptom management and encouraging healthy aging are revealed.

We acknowledge the influence of lifestyle variables on hormonal health, such as exercise, stress management, and sleep, as we wrap up our investigation. We unearth behaviors and practices that promote general well-being as well as hormonal balance.

The tale of hormonal balance plan for women is woven together from science, biology, and personal experience. It's a voyage that defies age and space, a celebration of the strength and beauty of women and their hormones. We are going to go on an adventure that honors the remarkable role that hormones play in our lives and provides women with the information and resources they need to accept and appreciate their unique hormonal makeup. This thorough handbook will lead us as we make our way through its chapters. Join us as we embrace this enthralling journey with all of its trials and victories and discover the keys to living a life in which hormonal balance is king.

Chapter 1

Understanding Women's Hormones

Hormones are essential for controlling many bodily physiological and psychological functions. The complex dance of hormone swings is an essential feature of women's biology in particular. Throughout her lifetime, a woman experiences these swings, which affect everything from her reproductive health to her mood and energy levels. The complexities of women's hormones, their functions, the several phases of a woman's life when they are most significant, and the effects of hormonal imbalances on a woman's general health will all be covered in-depth in this extensive book.

Basics of Women's Hormones

Hormones Defined

Endocrine system glands and organs create hormones, which are chemical messengers. They have certain target organs or tissues that they move via the circulation to affect. Estrogen, progesterone, and testosterone are important hormones for women, but many other hormones are equally vital to their general health.

Estrogen

The three main hormones that makeup estrogen are estrone, estradiol, and estriol. Although small quantities are also created in fat cells and the adrenal glands, the ovaries are the primary site of production. Numerous elements of female health are attributed to estrogen, such as controlling the menstrual cycle, promoting reproductive health, preserving bone density, and affecting mood and mental processes.

Progesterone

Another crucial hormone for women's health is progesterone, which is mostly produced in the ovaries. It is essential for preserving pregnancy and getting the uterine lining ready for implantation. Progesterone affects mood in addition to contributing to a relaxed sensation.

Testosterone

Although testosterone is often associated with males, women also generate less of it. It supports general vigor, libido, and the health of muscles and bones. Women who have an excess of testosterone in their bodies may have several health problems, such as PCOS.

The Menstrual Cycle

Phases of the Menstrual Cycle

The menstrual cycle, which varies from woman to woman, is a normal, cyclical process that lasts around 28 days. Menstruation, ovulation, the luteal phase, and the follicular phase are among its stages.

- **Menstruation:** Menstruation, or the loss of the uterine lining, is the first stage of the cycle. This often lasts three to seven days.

- **Follicular Phase:** This stage lasts from the conclusion of the menstrual cycle until ovulation. The body uses this period to stimulate the development of follicles in the ovaries in preparation for a possible pregnancy.

- **Ovulation:** A developed follicle releases an egg in the middle of the cycle, which sperm may fertilize. Usually, ovulation happens on day 14 of the cycle.

- **Luteal Phase:** The empty follicle develops into the corpus luteum, which secretes progesterone to aid in the possibility of a pregnancy, after ovulation. Progesterone levels fall and menstruation resumes if pregnancy is not achieved.

Hormonal Fluctuations during the Menstrual Cycle

The levels of progesterone and estrogen vary throughout the menstrual cycle. Estrogen predominates during the follicular phase, encouraging the uterine lining to develop and producing more cervical mucus. Progesterone takes over after ovulation, protecting the uterine lining and getting the body ready for pregnancy.

Comprehending these hormonal oscillations is crucial for anticipating and managing an extensive array of menstruation symptoms, such as mood swings, bloating, and libido shifts.

Puberty

Hormonal Changes During Puberty

In both boys and girls, puberty is marked by substantial hormonal changes that signal the passage from infancy to maturity. The increased synthesis of estrogen in females is the main cause of these alterations.

- **Breast Development:** The growth of breast tissue and the emergence of mammary glands are caused by estrogen's stimulation of breast development.

- **Menstruation:** The regular release of eggs by the ovaries marks the beginning of menstruation, also known as menarche. Typically, this occurs in the age range of 12 to 14.

- **Growth Spurts:** During puberty, estrogen also plays a role in the development of secondary sexual traits including broader hips and a larger proportion of body fat.

Emotional and Psychological Changes

A girl's emotional and psychological health might be impacted by hormonal changes that occur throughout puberty. Mood swings, impatience, and increased emotional sensitivity are prevalent during this period. Parents and teenagers can better manage the difficulties of puberty if they are aware of these changes.

<u>Pregnancy</u>

Hormonal Changes During Pregnancy

The amazing adventure of pregnancy is marked by significant hormonal changes. The primary hormones implicated are progesterone, estrogen, and human chorionic gonadotropin (hCG).

- **hCG:** The hormone released by the growing placenta and identified by pregnancy tests is hCG. The corpus luteum, which continues to generate progesterone to sustain the pregnancy, is maintained in part by its existence.

- **Estrogen and progesterone:** Throughout pregnancy, these hormones keep rising, promoting the fetus's growth and development, controlling the uterine environment, and getting the body ready for delivery and nursing.

Common Hormonal Pregnancy Symptoms

Hormonal shifts during pregnancy may cause a range of symptoms, including mood swings, changes in skin tone, and morning nausea. The dramatic fluctuations in hormone levels are a major cause of these symptoms.

Menopause

Menopause Defined

Menopause, which signifies the end of a woman's reproductive years, is a normal aspect of aging. It usually happens between 45 and 55 years of age, however, it may happen later or sooner (premature menopause).

Hormonal Changes During Menopause

The production of estrogen and progesterone declines throughout menopause, which is the most major hormonal shift. This is a slow process that may cause mood swings, libido fluctuations, hot flashes, and night sweats, among other symptoms. It can take years to complete.

Perimenopause

Perimenopause is the term for the transitional phase that precedes menopause. Hormone levels fluctuate throughout this time, resulting in irregular periods and a variety of symptoms. For women to effectively handle the physical and psychological difficulties associated with the perimenopausal era, understanding it is essential.

Hormonal Imbalances

Hormonal Imbalance Causes

A woman's health may be significantly impacted by hormonal abnormalities, which can happen at any point in her life. Numerous things, including stress, food preferences, drug use, and underlying medical disorders, may cause these imbalances.

Polycystic Ovary Syndrome (PCOS)

PCOS is a prevalent hormonal condition affecting fertile women. It may cause ovarian cysts, irregular periods, and other health problems. It is characterized by an imbalance of sex hormones, especially high amounts of testosterone.

Hormone Replacement Therapy (HRT)

A medical procedure called hormone replacement therapy uses supplements of progesterone and estrogen to address menopausal symptoms. Women who are suffering from severe menopausal symptoms may find it helpful, but the advantages and disadvantages must be carefully weighed.

Hormones and Women's Health

Bone Health

For bone density to be maintained, estrogen is essential. Osteoporosis risk and increased bone fragility might result from the decrease in estrogen levels that occurs after menopause. For women to take action to promote their bone health, they must understand this relationship.

Cardiovascular Health

Additionally, estrogen lowers the risk of heart disease and regulates cholesterol levels, which protects the cardiovascular system. Women must take proactive measures to maintain their heart health since the loss of estrogen after menopause might raise the risk of heart disease.

Mental Health

A woman's mental health might be impacted by changes in her hormones. Recognizing and successfully treating mood disorders, such as anxiety and depression, requires an understanding of the relationship between hormones and these ailments.

Managing Hormonal Health

Nutrition and Lifestyle

Hormone regulation and the likelihood of hormonal imbalances may be decreased by leading a healthy lifestyle that includes stress management, frequent exercise, and a balanced diet. Dietary decisions such as ingesting foods high in phytoestrogens may also help women's hormone health.

Medical Treatments

Medical treatments may be required in situations of severe hormonal abnormalities or medical diseases such as PCOS. These may consist of prescription drugs, hormone treatments, and operations. Women must speak with medical specialists to learn about individualized treatment plans.

Holistic Approaches

When it comes to managing their hormonal health, some women choose supplementary and holistic methods including herbal medicines, acupuncture, and mindfulness exercises. Even while they may not be the main course of therapy for hormone imbalances, they can be a helpful addition to traditional medical care.

For women of all ages, it is vital to comprehend women's hormones. Hormones affect several facets of physical, emotional, and mental health in addition to reproductive health. Women may take charge of their health and well-being by understanding the functions of important hormones, the periods of a woman's life when they are most significant, and how to treat hormonal imbalances. Equipped with information, women may support their lifelong hormonal health by making educated decisions regarding diet, lifestyle, and healthcare.

Chapter 2

Hormonal Imbalances

A major worry that may impact people of all ages and genders is hormonal imbalances. Numerous physiological processes are regulated by hormones, and disturbances in their levels may result in a host of health problems. The first step in treating these issues and obtaining the necessary medical attention is identifying the telltale signs and symptoms of hormone abnormalities.

Biochemical messengers and hormones are created by the body's endocrine glands. They are circulating in the circulation and are critical for controlling immunological response, growth, metabolism, reproduction, and mood, among other key processes. For general health and well-being, these hormones must be kept in a careful balance.

Thyroid, insulin, sex, and adrenal hormone abnormalities are among the common hormonal disorders. Hormones that regulate the body's metabolic rate, such as triiodothyronine (T3) and thyroxine (T4), are produced by the thyroid gland. Unexpected changes in weight, weariness, heart rate fluctuations, and mood swings are all indications of a thyroid hormone imbalance. Thyroid diseases include conditions like hypothyroidism, in which the thyroid is underactive, and a high level of in which the thyroid is hyperactive.

Blood glucose is regulated by the pancreatic hormone insulin. Diabetes, which is characterized by high blood sugar, may be brought on by imbalances. Diabetes may cause weariness, impaired eyesight, increased thirst, and frequent urination. Progesterone, estrogen, and testosterone are examples of sex hormones that are essential for reproductive health and general well-being. Sexual dysfunction, mood swings, irregular menstrual cycles, and reproductive troubles may all be caused by hormonal imbalances.

Hormones like cortisol, which aid the body's reaction to stress, are produced by the adrenal glands. Disorders such as Addison's disease (insufficient cortisol) and Cushing's syndrome (excess cortisol) may be caused by imbalances. Increased body weight, elevated blood pressure, and exhaustion are possible signs.

Women who have hormonal abnormalities often experience irregular menstruation. Hormonal imbalances are often shown by irregular periods, heavy or light flow, and skipped periods. Unexpected weight gain or loss may be a sign of hormonal imbalances, which are often connected to problems with the thyroid or insulin. Hormone levels and skin health are intimately related. Unbalanced hormones might cause dryness, excessive oiliness, or acne. Acne outbreaks may be brought on by elevated androgens, or male hormones.

Hormonal problems may be the cause of thinning hair or excessive hair growth in undesirable places. Unbalances in hormones, especially androgen-related ones, often cause these alterations. Hormonal changes have a big impact on mood stability. Hormonal mood swings include conditions such as Premenstrual Syndrome (PMS) and Premenstrual Dysphoric Disorder (PMDD). Sleep cycles are significantly influenced by hormones such as the stress hormone cortisol. Chronic tiredness and sleep difficulties may be caused by elevated cortisol levels. Insulin and cortisol are two hormones that have an impact on gut health. Constipation, diarrhea, and bloating are examples of digestive problems that may result from hormonal abnormalities.

Hormonal abnormalities, particularly low testosterone in both men and women, have been linked to a reduction in libido. Unbalances in thyroid hormones may impact blood pressure and heart rate. Low blood pressure and a slower heart rate are two symptoms of hypothyroidism. Menopause is often linked to hot flashes and nocturnal sweats since estrogen levels drop dramatically during this time. Hormonal imbalances may cause irregularities in the menstrual cycle and ovulation, which can make it difficult to conceive. Hormonal changes may cause cognitive alterations that affect everyday functioning, memory, and focus. Women with low estrogen levels are more likely to develop osteoporosis because of a decrease in bone density.

Unbalanced hormone levels have a significant effect on general health and well-being. They may cause more serious health issues if they are not treated. Addressing these issues requires more than just recognizing the telltale signs and symptoms of hormone abnormalities. Restoring hormonal balance and enhancing general health and well-being need accurate diagnosis and treatment. People may restore hormonal balance and enhance their general health and quality of life with medical intervention, lifestyle modifications, and, in some situations, hormone replacement therapy. To proactively treat these issues and achieve long-term well-being, one must have a thorough understanding of the complexity of hormone imbalances and their effects on health.

Chapter 3

Stress and Hormonal Harmony

Stress is a natural aspect of life and may have a big influence on hormone balance. The chemical messengers of the body, hormones control many physiological functions, including stress reactions. Stress may cause hormone imbalances that can impact both physical and mental health when it becomes severe or persistent. To offer a thorough grasp of the subject and management techniques for stress-induced hormone imbalances, this extensive book explores the intricate link between stress and hormonal equilibrium.

The Physiology of Stress

The Stress Response

One must first understand the body's stress response to grasp the relationship between stress and hormones. The brain starts a series of actions when it senses a stressor, either psychological or physical. Adrenocorticotropic hormone (ACTH) is released by the pituitary gland in response to signals from the brain's hypothalamus. The main stress hormone, cortisol, is then secreted by the adrenal glands in response to ACTH. Cortisol is released to prepare the body for the "fight or flight" response by raising blood pressure, and heart rate, and releasing stored energy. This adaptive reaction promotes survival under acute stress settings. On the other hand, severe or chronic stress may cause several health problems.

The Role of Cortisol

A key player in regulating hormone balance and the stress response is cortisol. It affects several physiological functions, such as blood sugar management, immunological response, and metabolism. Although prolonged or excessive cortisol production may result in hormone imbalances and health issues, cortisol is necessary for managing stress in the short term. High cortisol levels interfere with the synthesis of other hormones, including thyroid and insulin hormones, which may upset the balance of hormones.

The Impact of Chronic Stress on Hormonal Harmony

The HPA Axis Dysregulation

The hypothalamic-pituitary-adrenal (HPA) axis is a vital mechanism for stress response and hormonal balance, and chronic stress may disrupt this system. Extended periods of stress may cause the overproduction of cortisol, which suppresses the HPA axis and reduces reactivity. The hormonal balance may be upset by this, leading to a persistent condition of hypercortisolism marked by elevated cortisol levels. Other hormone systems, such as the thyroid and reproductive hormones, might suffer as a consequence.

Thyroid Hormone Disruption

The synthesis and control of thyroid hormones, which are vital for metabolism, energy balance, and general health, may be upset by prolonged stress. Reduced conversion of the inactive thyroid hormone thyroxine (T4) to the active form triiodothyronine (T3) might result from stress-induced alterations in the HPA axis. This may lead to hypothyroidism, which manifests as weariness, weight gain, and cognitive decline. Stress management is essential to maintaining hormonal balance and thyroid function.

Reproductive Hormone Imbalances

Stress may alter the balance of sex hormones, which can affect fertility and reproductive health. Prolonged stress in women may mess with their menstrual cycle, causing irregular periods or even amenorrhea (no menstruation). The hypothalamus and pituitary gland, which control the synthesis of sex hormones including progesterone and estrogen, may also be impacted by stress. Chronic stress in males may result in lower testosterone levels, which have an impact on sexual function and general health.

The Impact on Insulin and Blood Sugar Control

Elevations in cortisol brought on by stress may impact blood sugar regulation and insulin sensitivity. Insulin resistance, in which cells lose their sensitivity to insulin signals, may be brought on by persistently high cortisol levels. This can raise blood sugar levels. This plays a major role in the development of type 2 diabetes. Maintaining insulin sensitivity and promoting hormonal balance need effective stress management.

Emotional and Cognitive Consequences of Stress-Related Hormonal Imbalances

Mood and Mental Health

Hormonal imbalances brought on by stress may have a big impact on mental and emotional well-being. Anxiety and depressive symptoms may be brought on by high cortisol levels. In addition to affecting the synthesis of neurotransmitters like serotonin and dopamine, chronic stress may also cause mood changes. To treat diseases like anxiety and depression, it is essential to comprehend the relationship between stress, hormones, and mental health.

Cognitive Function

Chronic stress-related hormonal imbalances may affect how well the brain functions. Memory loss, focus issues, and difficulty making decisions may be caused by high cortisol levels. It's common to refer to this cognitive impairment as "brain fog." Understanding how hormone balance affects cognitive performance is essential for treating stress-related memory and cognitive problems.

Physical Health Implications

Cardiovascular Health

Persistent stress may damage cardiovascular health, mainly by throwing off the balance of hormones. Increased blood pressure, inflammation, and oxidative stress are all consequences of elevated cortisol levels, and they may play a role in the development of cardiovascular diseases such as hypertension, atherosclerosis, and heart disease. Maintaining cardiovascular health and lowering the risk of heart-related problems need effective stress management.

Gastrointestinal Health

Irritable bowel syndrome (IBS) and other gastrointestinal disorders may be brought on by stress, which can have a substantial impact on digestive health. Stress-related hormonal imbalances may affect the gut's permeability, motility, and microbial composition. Understanding how stress affects hormonal balance is crucial to treating digestive issues and fostering gastrointestinal health.

Immune Function

Hormonal homeostasis is closely related to the immune system. People who experience ongoing stress may have weakened immune systems, leaving them more vulnerable to infections and diseases. Prolonged elevation of cortisol may depress immune function and make it harder for the body to fight against infections. It is essential to comprehend the relationship between stress and the immune system to preserve general health.

Strategies for Restoring Hormonal Harmony and Managing Stress

Stress Management Techniques

Putting stress management strategies into practice is essential to reestablishing hormonal balance. These methods include gradual muscular relaxation, yoga, deep breathing exercises, and mindfulness meditation. The effects of chronic stress may be lessened and cortisol levels lowered by partaking in stress-relieving activities.

Regular Exercise

It has been shown that regular exercise lowers stress and supports hormonal equilibrium. Exercise releases endorphins, which are naturally occurring mood boosters. Moreover, exercise may enhance metabolic health and insulin sensitivity. Including regular exercise in one's routine is crucial for stress management and hormone balance.

Nutrition & Diet

Diet is essential for promoting hormonal balance and stress management. Foods high in nutrients, such as fruits, vegetables, whole grains, lean meats, and healthy fats, provide the body with the vital vitamins and minerals it needs to regulate hormones. Hormonal balance may also be achieved by consuming less processed and highly refined meals. Furthermore, certain meals might lessen the negative effects of long-term stress on the body, such as those high in antioxidants and omega-3 fatty acids.

Adequate Sleep

Stress reduction and hormonal balance depend heavily on sleep. Hormonal imbalances may result from inadequate sleep, particularly in cortisol and melatonin. Taking excellent care of oneself when it comes to sleep hygiene and adhering to a regular sleep pattern is crucial to regulating hormone imbalances brought on by stress.

Relationships and Social Support

Good connections and robust social support networks may serve as barriers against the negative consequences of stress. People may learn to manage stress and preserve their emotional health by keeping strong relationships with friends and family, asking for assistance when they need it, and encouraging pleasant social interactions.

Professional Help and Medication

Psychotherapy

When hormonal imbalances brought on by stress result in serious mental health problems such as depression and anxiety, psychotherapy, such as cognitive-behavioral therapy (CBT) or counseling, may be very beneficial. These treatment modalities assist people in building resilience and coping mechanisms so they can control their stress and preserve emotional equilibrium.

Medication

Medical intervention may be required in some cases to treat hormonal abnormalities brought on by stress. When emotional and mental health problems are severe and uncontrollable, doctors may prescribe drugs like antidepressants or anxiety pills. The best course of therapy must be determined after consulting with a healthcare provider.

Hormonal balance and stress have a complex and multidimensional interaction. Prolonged stress may cause hormone imbalances that impact one's physical, mental, and emotional health.

Comprehending the hormonal effects of stress is essential for managing a variety of health concerns, ranging from emotional dysregulation and cognitive deficits to cardiovascular diseases and digestive disorders. The significance of stress management techniques and lifestyle decisions that support emotional resilience, physical health, and hormonal balance is highlighted by the understanding of the intricate interactions between stress and hormones. In the end, hormone balance is a dynamic process that necessitates a comprehensive strategy that takes into account one's physical, mental, and nutritional health.

Chapter 4

The Menstrual Cycle

A complicated and normal biological process that affects people with reproductive systems is the menstrual cycle. It entails a complex set of monthly hormonal and physiological adjustments made in anticipation of a possible pregnancy. This in-depth manual attempts to explore the complexities of the menstrual cycle, including its stages, hormonal management, typical variances, and the role that this cycle plays in an individual's reproductive health.

Introduction to the Menstrual Cycle

Defining the Menstrual Cycle

For females of reproductive age, the menstrual cycle is a cyclical process that usually lasts for 28 days, however, there are some variances. Getting the body ready for a possible pregnancy requires several hormonal oscillations and physiological changes in the reproductive system. There are several stages to the cycle, and each is essential to the reproductive process.

Menarche and Puberty

Puberty, which usually lasts from the ages of 10 to 16, marks the beginning of the menstrual cycle and leads to menarche, or the start of menstruation. Menarche is the beginning of the menstrual cycle and the start of a person's capacity for reproduction.

Hormonal Regulation of the Menstrual Cycle

The Role of Hormones

The menstrual cycle is mostly controlled by hormones. A complicated interaction of hormones, mostly regulated by the pituitary, ovaries, and brain, orchestrates the cycle. Main hormones consist of:

Gonadotropin-Releasing Hormone (GnRH)

Gonadotropins are released by the pituitary gland in response to a signal from the brain called GnRH.

Follicle-Stimulating Hormone (FSH) and Luteinizing Hormone (LH)

FSH and LH, two gonadotropins secreted by the pituitary gland, drive follicle development in the ovaries and initiate ovulation and the formation of the corpus luteum, respectively.

Progesterone and estrogen

These hormones, which are produced by the ovaries, are vital for controlling the menstrual cycle. Progesterone supports a prospective pregnancy and aids in endometrial maintenance, whereas estrogen promotes the thickness of the uterine lining (endometrium).

Phases of the Menstrual Cycle

There are many stages to the menstrual cycle:

- **Menstrual Phase:** The cycle starts with menstruation, which is followed by the evacuation of tissue and blood as a result of the uterine lining being lost. Usually, this stage lasts three to seven days.

- **Follicular Phase:** The follicular phase starts after menstruation. An immature egg is contained in each ovarian follicle that grows as a result of FSH stimulation. As estrogen levels increase, the endometrium thickens in anticipation of the possible implantation of a fertilized egg.

- **Ovulation:** Ovulation is brought on by a rise in LH midway through the cycle, usually around day 14 in a 28-day cycle. An egg (ovum), which is ready for fertilization, is released from the ovary into the fallopian tube when the mature follicle bursts.

- **Luteal Phase:** The residual follicle develops into the corpus luteum, which secretes progesterone, after ovulation. To prepare the endometrium for possible embryo implantation, this hormone maintains it. The cycle restarts if fertilization is unsuccessful because the corpus luteum degrades and progesterone levels fall.

Variations and Characteristics of the Menstrual Cycle

Menstrual Irregularities

Menstrual cycles vary from person to person and are impacted by several variables, including:

- **Cycle Length:** Variations are typical, although the average cycle lasts around 28 days. Cycle lengths vary from 21 to 35 days, with slight fluctuations occurring every month.

- **Time and Volume of Bleeding:** The duration of menstrual bleeding may vary from two to seven days, with a mild to heavy flow.

- **Pain and Symptoms:** Premenstrual syndrome (PMS) may cause discomfort in the form of cramps, bloating, mood swings, and soreness in the breasts. Severe symptoms might be a sign of

PMDD, or premenstrual dysphoric disorder.

Menstrual Disorders

Some anomalies in menstruation may be a sign of underlying medical conditions:

- **Amenorrhea:** is the absence of menstruation. It may be primary (not starting at age 15) or secondary (not starting at all in a person who was previously consistently menstruating for at least three months).

- **Dysmenorrhea:** A painful menstrual cycle, usually brought on by contractions in the uterus.

- **Menorrhagia:** Prolonged or excessive menstrual bleeding, which may be a sign of anatomical defects or hormonal imbalances.

Reproductive Health and the Menstrual Cycle

Fertility and Conception

It is essential for anyone attempting to conceive to understand the menstrual cycle. The best window of time for conception is the fertile window, which is the period before and after ovulation. For people trying conception, monitoring the menstrual cycle might help determine the most fertile days.

Pregnancy and Menstrual Cycle

The menstrual cycle is upset during pregnancy. Hormonal changes brought on by the fertilized egg implanting in the uterine lining after fertilization stop menstruation. The major indication of pregnancy is the lack of menstruation.

Menstrual Hygiene and Management

Hygiene Practices

Reproductive health depends on practicing good menstrual hygiene.

Menstrual flow may be controlled and infections can be avoided by using sanitary goods such as pads, tampons, menstrual cups, or period underwear. To lower the chance of bacterial development, it's important to replace sanitary items regularly.

Pain Management

Many people suffer from pain or cramping during their menstruation. Menstrual discomfort may be managed with over-the-counter painkillers, heating pads, and lifestyle modifications including exercise and a balanced diet.

Menstruation in Cultural and Societal Contexts

Cultural Perceptions

Menstruation is seen differently by cultures all across the globe. Menstruating people are occasionally stigmatized or subjected to prejudice because of the many customs, taboos, and beliefs that exist in many communities. To debunk misconceptions and advance good views toward menstruation, activism, and education are essential.

Access to Menstrual Health Resources

Global access to resources for menstruation health, such as education, sanitary napkins, and appropriate medical treatment, is a challenge. Menstruating people have difficulties across the globe due to restricted access to menstrual hygiene products and insufficient knowledge about reproductive health.

An essential component of reproductive health is the menstrual cycle, which indicates the body's preparedness for possible conception. Comprehending its stages, hormonal control, fluctuations, and importance is crucial for the general health and welfare of humans. Promoting reproductive health and fostering a welcoming atmosphere for those going through menstruation include pushing for better resources for menstrual health, educating people about their menstrual cycles, and resolving abnormalities. Recognizing and honoring the menstrual cycle promotes the physical and mental health of people everywhere by enabling them to accept this essential feature of existence.

Chapter 5

Hormonal Balance Through Nutrition

Hormonal balance affects many body processes and general health, making it a crucial component of well-being. One cannot emphasize how important diet is to preserving and enhancing hormonal health. We will look at how various meals might be adapted to assist hormonal balance throughout the day in this extensive guide. Hormone-friendly nighttime meals, hormone-fueling breakfasts, and hormone-balancing morning lunches—every meal provides a chance to support hormonal equilibrium.

<u>Breakfast</u>

Mornings set the tone for the rest of the day, so start your day off right with a hormone-balancing breakfast that gives your body the critical nutrients it needs to stay healthy.

1. Avocado and Egg Breakfast Wrap

Ingredients:

- 1/4 cup diced tomatoes

- 1 whole-grain or spinach tortilla

- 2 large eggs, scrambled

- 1 ripe avocado, mashed

- Salt and pepper to taste

- Fresh cilantro or parsley for garnish

Preparation:

Mash the avocado and place it on a whole-grain or spinach tortilla to make the Avocado and Egg Breakfast Wrap. Two big eggs should be scrambled and topped with the avocado. Once the tomatoes are chopped, add some salt and pepper to taste. Add some fresh parsley or cilantro as a garnish. Enjoy this hormone-balancing breakfast wrap by rolling up the tortilla, cutting it in half, and eating it.

2. Berry Bliss Smoothie Bowl

Ingredients:

- 1 cup mixed berries (strawberries, blueberries, raspberries)

- 1 tablespoon chia seeds

- 1/4 cup rolled oats

- 1/2 cup Greek yogurt

- 1 tablespoon honey

- Fresh mint leaves for garnish

Preparation:

Blend the mixed berries, Greek yogurt, rolled oats, chia seeds, and honey in a blender until the mixture is smooth and creamy to make the Berry Bliss Smoothie Bowl. Transfer the blended drink to a dish and top with more fresh berries, chia seeds, and fresh mint leaves. This tasty and nourishing dish is the ideal way to start your day with hormones in balance.

3. Fruit and Chia Seed Pudding

Ingredients:

- 1/2 teaspoon vanilla extract

- 2 tablespoons chia seeds

- Half a cup almond milk (or any other kind of milk you choose)

- Honey or maple syrup for drizzling

- Fresh mixed fruit (e.g., sliced kiwi, strawberries, and blueberries)

Preparation:

In a dish, combine chia seeds, almond milk, and vanilla essence to make Chia Seed Pudding with Fresh Fruit. After giving the mixture a good stir to make sure the chia seeds are firmly submerged, cover and chill it for at least three hours or overnight. Drizzle honey or maple syrup over the fresh mixed fruit on top of the chia pudding in the morning. This filling pudding makes a tasty, hormone-balancing breakfast.

4. Spinach and Mushroom Breakfast Quesadilla

Ingredients:

- 2 whole-grain tortillas

- 1/2 cup sliced mushrooms

- 1 cup fresh spinach

- 1/4 cup shredded mozzarella cheese

- 2 eggs, scrambled

- Olive oil for cooking

- Salt and pepper to taste

Preparation:

To make the breakfast quesadilla with spinach and mushrooms, heat some olive oil in a pan over medium heat. Add the fresh spinach and heat until it wilts after sautéing the sliced mushrooms until they become brown. After taking out the veggies from the pan, use it to scramble two eggs. Add pepper and salt for seasoning. Layer shredded mozzarella cheese, sautéed veggies, and scrambled eggs on top of one tortilla that has been placed in the pan. After the first tortilla is golden brown on all sides, place the second one on top. Take a bite out of the quesadilla and enjoy your hormone-balancing breakfast.

5. Pancake with Banana Nuts

Ingredients:

- 2 eggs

- 1/4 cup chopped walnuts

- 1 ripe banana, mashed

- A pinch of cinnamon

- Olive oil for cooking (or cooking spray)

Preparation:

In a bowl, mix the mashed banana, eggs, chopped walnuts, and a dash of cinnamon to make Banana Nut Pancakes. Apply frying spray or olive oil to a nonstick pan to get it hot. Spoon tiny dollops of the batter into the skillet, and cook until golden brown on both sides. For a delicious and hormone-balancing breakfast, top your banana nut pancakes with a drizzle of honey or a dollop of Greek yogurt.

6. Greek Yogurt Parfait

Ingredients:

- 1/4 cup granola

- 1 cup Greek yogurt

- Mixed berries (e.g., strawberries, blueberries, and raspberries)

- Honey for drizzling

Preparation:

To make the Greek Yogurt Parfait, fill a glass or dish with layers of Greek yogurt, granola, and mixed berries. Pour honey over top, then keep layering and drizzling as you want. A satisfying and healthy way to start the day with a hormone-balancing breakfast is with this parfait.

7. Blueberry and Almond Overnight Oats

Ingredients:

- 1/2 cup rolled oats

- 1 tablespoon almond butter

- Honey for drizzling

- 1 cup almond milk

- 1/4 cup fresh blueberries

- Sliced almonds for topping

Preparation:

Rolling oats and almond milk should be combined in a jar or other container to create Almond and Blueberry, Overnight Oats. A dab of almond butter and fresh blueberries should be added. Pour some honey on top. Once the container is sealed, chill it for the whole night. Sprinkle sliced almonds on top in the morning, then eat your hormone-balancing overnight oats.

Lunch

Lunch is a chance to replenish your body's energy and make sure your hormones are getting the nourishment they need to work at their best.

1. Salad with Lentils and Spinach

Ingredients:

- 1/4 cup sliced red onion

- 1 cup cooked green or brown lentils

- 1/2 cup crumbled feta cheese

- 2 cups fresh spinach

- 1/4 cup cherry tomatoes, halved

- Salt and pepper to taste

- 2 tablespoons balsamic vinaigrette

Preparation:

In a salad bowl, mix cooked lentils, fresh spinach, feta cheese crumbles, cherry tomatoes, and sliced red onion for the Lentil and Spinach Salad. After drizzling the salad with the balsamic vinaigrette, toss to coat. Season with pepper and salt to taste. For a delicious and healthy meal that balances hormones, try this salad.

2. Stuffed Bell Peppers with Quinoa

Ingredients:

- 1/4 cup chopped fresh cilantro

- 4 bell peppers (assorted colors)

- 1 cup diced tomatoes

- 1 cup of corn kernels (frozen, or canned, fresh,)

- 1 cup cooked quinoa

- 1 teaspoon cumin

- 1 can black beans, drained and rinsed

- Salt and pepper to taste

Preparation:

Remove the seeds and chop off the tops of the bell peppers for the Quinoa Stuffed Bell Peppers. Black beans, corn kernels, diced tomatoes, chopped cilantro, cumin, cooked quinoa, and salt and pepper should all be combined in a dish. Place the quinoa mixture into the bell peppers. After putting the filled bell peppers in a baking dish and covering it with foil, bake them for 25 to 30 minutes at 375°F (190°C), or until they are soft. Serve these tasty and vibrant stuffed peppers for a hormone-balancing midday meal.

3. Vegetable and Grilled Chicken Bowl

Ingredients:

- 2 cloves garlic, minced

- 2 boneless, skinless chicken breasts

- 1 zucchini, sliced

- 1 red bell pepper, sliced

- 2 tablespoons olive oil

- 2 cups broccoli florets

- Lemon wedges

- Fresh herbs for garnish (e.g., basil or parsley)

- Salt and pepper to taste

Preparation:

To make the Grilled Chicken and Vegetable Bowl, drizzle some olive oil over the chicken breasts, broccoli, red bell pepper, and zucchini. Add salt, pepper, and minced garlic to the chicken and veggies for seasoning. The chicken and veggies should be cooked through and have a hint of sear on the grill. Cut the chicken into thin pieces. Present the grilled chicken and veggies in a dish with lemon wedges and fresh herb garnishes. This well-balanced meal is full of nutrients that are good for hormones.

4. Black bean and Quinoa Salad

Ingredients:

- 1 cup cherry tomatoes, halved

- 1 cup cooked quinoa

- 1 can black beans, drained and rinsed

- 1/4 cup chopped fresh cilantro

- Juice of 1 lime

- 1 cup diced bell peppers (assorted colors)

- 2 tablespoons olive oil

- Salt and pepper to taste

Preparation:

To make the Quinoa and Black Bean Salad, fill a large bowl with cooked quinoa, black beans, chopped cilantro, sliced bell peppers, and cherry tomatoes. To make the dressing, combine the lime juice, olive oil, salt, and pepper in another bowl. Over the salad, drizzle with the dressing and toss to mix. Enjoy a hormone-balancing meal while serving cold.

5. Salmon and Asparagus Foil Packets

Ingredients:

- 2 cloves garlic, minced

- 2 tablespoons olive oil

- Fresh dill for garnish

- 2 salmon fillets

- 1 bunch of asparagus

- Lemon slices

- Salt and pepper to taste

Preparation:

Set oven temperature to 375°F (190°C) for Salmon and Asparagus Foil packet preparation. Every salmon fillet should be placed on a piece of aluminum foil. Place spears of asparagus around the salmon. Add a drizzle of olive oil and season with salt, pepper, and chopped garlic. Add fresh dill and lemon slices to the top of each package. After sealing the foil packets, bake the salmon for 15 to 20 minutes, or until it flakes easily. After serving the foil packets, enjoy your meal that balances hormones.

6. Curry with Chickpeas and Spinach

Ingredients:

- 1 can diced tomatoes

- 1 can chickpeas, drained and rinsed

- 2 cups fresh spinach

- 2 cloves garlic, minced

- 1 onion, finely chopped

- 1 can of coconut milk

- Salt and pepper to taste

- 2 tablespoons curry powder

- Cooked brown rice or whole-grain naan bread

Preparation:

To make the Chickpea and Spinach Curry, preheat a big skillet and sauté the minced garlic and chopped onion until they become transparent. After adding the curry powder, simmer for one more minute. Add coconut milk, chopped tomatoes, and chickpeas by stirring. Simmer for ten to fifteen minutes to let the flavors combine. Cook the fresh spinach till it wilts by adding it. Season with pepper and salt to taste. For a tasty and hormone-balancing lunch, serve the curry made with chickpeas and spinach over cooked brown rice or with whole-grain naan bread.

7. Stir-fried Broccoli and Tofu

Ingredients:

- 1 carrot, sliced

- 1 block extra-firm tofu, cubed

- 2 tablespoons low-sodium soy sauce

- 2 cups broccoli florets

- 1 red bell pepper, sliced

- 2 cloves garlic, minced

- Sesame seeds for garnish

- 1 tablespoon sesame oil

- Cooked brown rice

Preparation:

Heat the sesame oil in a large pan or wok over medium-high heat for the Tofu and Broccoli Stir-Fry. Stir-fry the cubed tofu until it begins to take on light brown hues. After removing, put the tofu aside. Stir-fry the carrot, red bell pepper, broccoli, and minced garlic in the same skillet until they are crisp-tender. After a few more minutes, add low-sodium soy sauce to the skillet with the tofu and cook it some longer. Serve with sesame seeds as a topping over cooked brown rice. A filling and hormone-balancing meal is this stir-fry.

These lunch ideas for balancing hormones provide a selection of delectable and healthy choices to enhance hormonal health and general well-being. Take pleasure in cooking and enjoying these dishes as a healthy component of your diet.

<u>Dinner</u>

Dinner is an opportunity to relax and fuel your body with suppertime foods that promote relaxation and renewal and are hormone-friendly.

1. Avocado and Shrimp Salad

Ingredients:

1/4 cup red onion, finely chopped

2 cups mixed greens

Fresh cilantro for garnish

1 lb shrimp, peeled and deveined

2 avocados, diced

2 tablespoons olive oil

Juice of 1 lime

Salt and pepper to taste

Preparation:

To prepare the Shrimp and Avocado Salad, place a pan over medium heat with olive oil. The shrimp should be sautéed until pink and opaque. The cooked shrimp, diced avocados, chopped red onion, and mixed greens should all be combined in a big salad dish. Pour in some lime juice and stir lightly. To taste, add salt and pepper for seasoning. Enjoy this hormone-balancing and light supper while garnished with freshly chopped cilantro.

2. Chickpea Curry and Eggplant

Ingredients:

- 1 can diced tomatoes

- 1 can of coconut milk

- 1 large eggplant, diced

- 2 cloves garlic, minced

- 1 can chickpeas, drained and rinsed

- 2 tablespoons curry powder

- Salt and pepper to taste

- Fresh cilantro for garnish

- Cooked brown rice or whole-grain naan bread

Preparation:

In a large skillet, sauté the diced eggplant and minced garlic until the eggplant is soft, about 3 minutes, to prepare the eggplant and chickpea curry. Cook for one more minute after adding the curry powder. Add the chopped tomatoes, coconut milk, and chickpeas. In order for the flavors to combine, simmer for ten to fifteen minutes. Add pepper and salt for seasoning. Garnish the eggplant and chickpea curry with fresh cilantro and serve it with whole-grain naan bread or cooked brown rice. Dinner with this aromatic curry is filling and hormone-balancing.

3. Grilled Chicken with Asparagus and Quinoa

Ingredients:

- 1 cup cooked quinoa

- 2 cloves garlic, minced

- 2 boneless, skinless chicken breasts

- 1 bunch asparagus

- 2 tablespoons olive oil

- Lemon wedges

- Fresh basil for garnish

- Salt and pepper to taste

Preparation:
Brush the asparagus and chicken breasts with olive oil to make Grilled Chicken with Quinoa and Asparagus. Add salt, pepper, and chopped garlic to season them. Cook the chicken and asparagus on the grill until they are well done and have lovely sear marks. Serve the chicken with grilled asparagus and cooked quinoa, sliced into strips. Dinner will be tasty and hormone-balancing if you garnish it with fresh basil and serve with lemon wedges.

4. Baked Salmon with Roasted Vegetables

Ingredients:

- 2 cloves garlic, minced

- 2 tablespoons olive oil

- 2 salmon fillets

- 2 cups mixed vegetables (e.g., broccoli, carrots, and bell peppers)

- Lemon wedges

- Fresh dill for garnish

- Salt and pepper to taste

Preparation:

Set your oven to 375°F (190°C) to bake the salmon with roasted vegetables. Spread the mixed veggies on a baking sheet after tossing them with olive oil, minced garlic, salt, and pepper. Place the salmon fillets over the veggies after seasoning with salt and pepper. Garnish with lemon wedges for taste. Bake for about 20 to 25 minutes, or until the veggies are soft and the salmon flakes easily. Serve this hormone-balancing, nutrient-rich supper with a fresh dill garnish.

5. Sweet Potato and Black Bean Bowl

Ingredients:

- 1/4 cup salsa

- 2 medium sweet potatoes, cubed

- 2 tablespoons olive oil

- 1 can black beans, drained and rinsed

- 2 cups fresh spinach

- 1/4 cup plain Greek yogurt

- Chili powder, cumin, and paprika for seasoning

- Salt and pepper to taste

Preparation:

To make the Sweet Potato and Black Bean Bowl, combine the sweet potato cubes with olive oil, cumin, paprika, chili powder, salt, and pepper. Roast them for 20 to 25 minutes, or until they are soft, at 400°F (200°C). Arrange roasted sweet potatoes, black beans, and fresh spinach in a serving dish. Add some salsa and a dollop of plain Greek yogurt on top. Dinner is a tasty, hormone-balancing dish of nutrients.

6. Vegetable and Stir-Fry Turkey

Ingredients:

- 1 red bell pepper, sliced

- 2 cloves garlic, minced

- Sesame seeds for garnish

- 1 lb ground turkey

- 2 cups broccoli florets

- 1 cup snap peas

- 2 tablespoons low-sodium soy sauce

- 1 tablespoon sesame oil

- Cooked brown rice

Preparation:

Sesame oil should be heated over medium-high heat in a big pan or wok for the Turkey and Vegetable Stir-Fry. When the ground turkey is browned, add it and simmer. Take out and place the turkey aside. Stir-fry the broccoli, red bell pepper, snap peas, and chopped garlic in the same skillet until they become crisp-tender. After adding the low-sodium soy sauce and returning the turkey to the pan, heat everything through for a few more minutes. Overcooked brown rice, serve this high-protein stir-fry and sprinkle with sesame seeds. Savor this delectable supper that balances hormones.

These tasty and nourishing hormone-balancing supper dishes provide a range of alternatives to promote general well-being and hormonal health. Take pleasure in cooking and enjoying these dishes as a healthy component of your diet.

7. Quinoa and Chickpea Stir-Fry

Ingredients:

- 2 cups broccoli florets

- 1 cup cooked quinoa

- 2 tablespoons low-sodium soy sauce

- 1 can chickpeas, drained and rinsed

- 1 red bell pepper, sliced

- 2 cloves garlic, minced

- 1 tablespoon sesame oil

- Sesame seeds for garnish

Preparation:

Heat the sesame oil in a large pan or wok over medium-high heat for the Quinoa and Chickpea Stir-Fry. Add the minced garlic, red bell pepper, and broccoli and sauté until they are crisp-tender. Add the chickpeas, low-sodium soy sauce, and cooked quinoa. Stir-fry for a further few minutes to allow the flavors to mingle. Add some sesame seeds as a garnish and serve this hormone-balancing, high-protein supper.

Incorporating these hormone-balancing meals into your daily routine can have a significant impact on your overall well-being. By understanding the importance of nutrients, balanced meals, and mindful eating, you can support your hormones and enjoy better health and vitality. Whether it's a hormone-balancing morning, a nourishing lunch, or a hormone-friendly evening meal, each meal offers an opportunity to promote hormonal harmony and well-being.

Chapter 6

Hormones and Weight Management

The complex interaction between hormones and weight control has many facets and has a significant impact on a person's capacity to reach and maintain a healthy weight. As the body's chemical messengers, hormones control a wide range of physiological functions, such as hunger, metabolism, and fat storage. Gaining an understanding of hormones' function in weight management is essential to creating methods that support weight reduction, maintenance, and general health. This thorough guide examines methods that help healthy weight control by focusing on establishing hormonal balance.

Hormones and Their Role in Weight Management

Insulin: The Blood Sugar Regulator
The pancreas secretes insulin, which is essential for controlling blood sugar levels. It makes glucose easier for cells to absorb and utilize as energy. High-glycemic meals may cause blood sugar rises and the consequent release of insulin. Knowing how insulin

functions in weight control is essential since food choices have a big influence on it.

Leptin: The Hormone of Satiety

The "satiety hormone," leptin, is generated by fat cells and controls hunger and body weight. When the body has enough energy reserves, it sends a signal to the brain to stop eating more. However, obesity may cause leptin resistance, a condition in which the brain is unable to process the hormone that causes appetite.

Ghrelin: The Hormone of Hunger

The "hunger hormone," ghrelin, is produced in the stomach and increases appetite. Before meals, its levels increase, and after eating, they decline.

Ghrelin production is highly influenced by meal time and selection, making it a crucial hormone to maintain weight.

Peptide YY (PYY): The Appetite Suppressor

The digestive system releases PYY mainly in reaction to the ingestion of fat and protein. It encourages decreased food intake and feelings of fullness. Setting aside meals that are high in protein and good fats will encourage PYY release, which helps with hunger management.

Cortisol: The Stress Hormone

The "stress hormone," cortisol, affects how people eat. Stress causes the body to produce more cortisol, which often increases appetite, particularly for comfort foods that are heavy in calories. Stress reduction strategies are crucial for controlling cortisol levels and encouraging better eating practices.

Strategies for Achieving Hormonal Balance

Balanced Macronutrients

Hormonal equilibrium must be supported by eating a diet of healthy fats, proteins, and carbs in appropriate amounts. Appetite, energy expenditure, and insulin responses are all regulated by a balanced diet. It is beneficial to metabolic health to prioritize whole grains, lean proteins, and healthy fats in regular meals.

Whole Foods and Nutrient Density

To sustain hormonal balance, it is essential to emphasize entire meals, such as fruits, vegetables, whole grains, lean meats, and healthy fats. Whole foods are high in nutrients and provide vital vitamins and minerals that help control hormones. Lowering the intake of highly refined and processed meals may improve general health.

Mindful Eating

Eating mindfully is being aware of your hunger signals, taking your time, and enjoying every meal. This method assists people in choosing more fulfilling and thoughtful foods. People who are in touch with their bodies can control their hormone reactions and promote a balanced diet.

Stress Management

Stress-reduction tactics, such as deep breathing exercises, relaxation methods, and meditation, assist in lowering cortisol levels and guard against hormone imbalances brought on by stress. Supporting good eating habits and general health requires lowering stress and preserving emotional stability.

Regular Meal Timing

Meal timing should be consistent to maintain a balanced hormonal response to meals by controlling the release of hormones. Timing meals consistently helps regulate hunger and maintain steady blood sugar levels.

Impact of Weight Management Strategies on Hormonal Balance

Low-Carb Diets

Low-carb diets, like Atkins or ketogenic diets, encourage fat-burning and lower insulin levels, which affect hormonal balance. These diets have the potential to be beneficial for weight reduction, especially for those who are insulin-resistant. It's crucial to keep in mind that they may not be appropriate for everyone and that their long-term consequences on hormone balance and general health need to be carefully considered.

Intermittent Fasting

The eating pattern of intermittent fasting, which consists of long intervals without meals interspersed with set eating windows, has a profound effect on the hormone reactions to food. Insulin levels drop during fasting, and the body starts using fat reserves for energy instead. Increased fat-burning and better insulin sensitivity are linked to this metabolic change. An efficient weight-management tactic might be intermittent fasting.

Plant-Based Diets

Hormone balance may benefit from plant-based diets, especially ones that are rich in whole foods and low in processed foods. Generally speaking, these diets are high in fiber, which helps control insulin and blood sugar levels. Furthermore, there is a correlation between reduced inflammation and a decreased likelihood of chronic illnesses and plant-based diets, which may have a favorable effect on hormonal balance and weight control.

Medical Interventions and Hormonal Therapy

Bariatric Surgery

A medical procedure for extreme obesity that results in significant weight reduction is bariatric surgery. Modifying gastrointestinal hormones that control hunger and metabolism, also affects hormonal balance. It has been shown that procedures like gastric bypass and sleeve gastrectomy lower ghrelin levels, boost PYY synthesis, and enhance insulin sensitivity.

Hormone Replacement Therapy (HRT)

Hormone replacement treatment may be recommended in some circumstances to treat hormonal abnormalities that impact weight control. For instance, HRT may be beneficial in supporting hormonal balance and metabolic health in those with thyroid diseases or polycystic ovarian syndrome (PCOS). A healthcare provider should be consulted before using HRT.

Comprehending the complex relationship between hormones and controlling weight is essential to general health and wellness. Hormones have a major impact on how the body processes food and reacts to it, affecting hunger, metabolism, and total weight. By understanding the functions of insulin, leptin, ghrelin, PYY, and cortisol, people may control their hunger, encourage appropriate weight management, and enhance their general well-being. A key component of individualized nutrition and health management is achieving hormonal balance through deliberate dietary and lifestyle decisions. This emphasizes the significant impact that these decisions have on hormonal balance and metabolic health.

Chapter 7

Aging Gracefully

Embracing the inevitable changes that come with age and figuring out how to keep our health and well-being are key components of aging gracefully. The hormonal changes that occur in women throughout menopause and perimenopause are an important part of aging. Our general quality of life may be significantly improved by being aware of these changes and putting methods in place to control symptoms and encourage healthy aging.

In women, menopause is a normal biological process that usually happens between the ages of 45 and 55. The absence of menstruation for a minimum of 12 consecutive months signifies the end of the reproductive years. But perimenopause—the period just before menopause—is just as significant and may last for several years. Hormonal changes start to happen during perimenopause, which results in a variety of mental and physical changes.

The two major female hormones, progesterone, and estrogen, are produced less often throughout menopause and perimenopause, and this is one of the fundamental hormonal changes that occurs during these phases.

These hormones are essential for controlling several body processes, such as the menstrual cycle, bone density, and mood swings. Many symptoms, including vaginal dryness, mood swings, hot flashes, and night sweats, might be brought on by a drop in hormone levels.

A multifaceted strategy is necessary to manage these symptoms and support healthy aging throughout perimenopause and menopause. The following techniques will be useful:

Hormone Replacement Therapy (HRT)

Hormone replacement therapy (HRT) uses pharmaceuticals to replenish the body's depleting progesterone and estrogen levels. It may enhance general well-being and lessen menopausal symptoms. Before contemplating HRT, however, it's crucial to speak with a healthcare provider since it may not be appropriate for everyone. They can help you make an educated choice by advising you on the possible advantages and disadvantages of HRT.

Lifestyle modifications

Modifying one's lifestyle in certain ways may help manage menopausal symptoms and encourage healthy aging. It is quite important to exercise regularly throughout this period. Exercise, such as yoga, swimming, or brisk walking, may enhance mood, preserve bone health, and lessen the intensity and frequency of hot flashes.

In addition, general health and well-being depend on eating a balanced diet rich in a range of fruits, vegetables, whole grains, lean meats, and healthy fats. Hormonal changes during menopause can cause weight gain, which may be managed with a balanced diet. Deep breathing exercises, meditation, and taking up hobbies are examples of stress-reduction strategies that may help reduce mood fluctuations and enhance mental health. Hormonal changes may cause sleep habits to be disrupted, therefore it's also essential to prioritize excellent sleep hygiene. A regular sleep schedule, a cozy sleeping environment, and abstaining from stimulants like coffee may all help to enhance sleep and lessen insomnia.

Natural remedies

Using natural therapies, some women experience relief from the symptoms associated with menopause. Some women have reported relief from symptoms using herbal supplements such as black cohosh, evening primrose oil, or phytoestrogens found in soy products. Before beginning any natural therapies, it's crucial to speak with a healthcare provider, however, since they can have negative effects or interfere with other prescriptions. Based on your unique medical circumstances, your healthcare practitioner may provide advice on how to utilize natural therapies appropriately.

Regular health check-ups

It is more important for women to prioritize routine health checkups as they age. This includes examinations of cardiovascular health, bone density tests to determine the risk of osteoporosis, and screenings for breast and cervical cancer. By monitoring your general health regularly, healthcare professionals can identify any possible problems early on and, if required, take the proper steps to address them. Keeping a positive rapport with your healthcare practitioner guarantees that you may get timely answers to any queries or issues you may have.

Emotional support and self-care

Emotionally, menopause may be a difficult period. It's crucial to ask for help from friends, family, or support groups so that you may exchange stories and learn from others who are traveling similar paths. In addition, sustaining emotional well-being requires engaging in self-care activities. Throughout menopause and beyond, making time for hobbies, rest, and introspection may help lower stress, elevate mood, and improve general quality of life.

To age gracefully, one must accept the hormonal changes that accompany menopause and perimenopause and develop coping mechanisms to reduce symptoms and encourage good aging. Important milestones in this path include comprehending the changes in hormone levels and making lifestyle adjustments, thinking about hormone replacement medication, investigating alternative therapies, making frequent health check-ups a priority, getting emotional support, and engaging in self-care. Keep in mind that every person's experience with menopause and aging is different, so it's important to pay attention to your body, make self-care a priority, and seek the advice of medical specialists for specific advice. You may maximize your general well-being and go through this stage of life with grace by being proactive.

Chapter 8

Lifestyle Factors for Hormonal Harmony

One of the most important aspects of general health and well-being is achieving hormonal equilibrium. Hormones act as messengers in the body, controlling several aspects of physiological processes. Lifestyle choices have a significant impact on hormone balance, impacting not just mood and energy levels but also metabolism and reproductive health.

This thorough book explores the major lifestyle elements that affect hormone balance, including how sleep, stress management, nutrition, exercise, and other factors affect hormonal balance and how to achieve and maintain optimum hormonal balance.

Diet and Nutrition

Balanced Diet for Hormonal Health

Hormonal balance starts with a well-balanced diet. Eating a wide variety of meals high in nutrients, such as whole grains, lean meats, healthy fats, and a bounty of fruits and vegetables, supplies vital vitamins and minerals that are important for hormone balance. Certain minerals that support hormonal balance and general health include zinc, magnesium, vitamin D, and omega-3 fatty acids.

Sugar and Hormonal Health

Consuming too much sugar may cause insulin to surge and then plummet, which can upset the balance of hormones. Consuming too much sugar is associated with insulin resistance, a disorder that impacts hormone balance and may result in obesity and other health problems. Hormonal balance may be enhanced by reducing intake of refined sugar and using natural sweeteners instead.

Impact of Caffeine and Alcohol

Alcohol and caffeine use may have an impact on hormone levels. While small amounts of coffee may not have a major negative impact on hormone balance, large amounts may raise cortisol levels and cause sleep disturbances, which can upset hormonal balance. Additionally, alcohol affects the metabolism and synthesis of hormones, especially on the balance of reproductive hormones.

Physical Activity and Exercise

Exercise and Hormonal Balance

Hormonal health is significantly impacted by regular physical exercise. Exercise lowers cortisol levels, increases the release of endorphins, or "feel-good" chemicals, and helps control insulin sensitivity. It has been shown that resistance and aerobic exercise both favorably impact hormone balance and general well-being.

Impact of Sedentary Lifestyle

Sedentary behavior might throw hormone balance off. Extended periods of inactivity and inactivity may result in weight gain, elevated cortisol levels, and impaired insulin sensitivity, all of which can have a detrimental impact on hormonal balance. Hormonal balance may be maintained by including frequent movement breaks and aiming for an active lifestyle.

Stress Management and Emotional Well-Being

Stress and Hormonal Imbalance

Hormonal equilibrium is greatly impacted by ongoing stress. Prolonged stress may raise cortisol levels, which can upset the body's chemical balance. Persistent stress may disrupt the hypothalamic-pituitary-adrenal (HPA) axis, resulting in hormone imbalances that impact mood, sleep quality, and general health.

Techniques for Stress Reduction

Chronic stress's negative effects on hormonal health may be lessened by engaging in stress-reduction practices including yoga, deep breathing exercises, mindfulness, meditation, and other relaxation techniques. Hormonal balance requires that you participate in activities that support mental health and relaxation.

Sleep and Hormonal Health

The Importance of Quality Sleep
Hormonal balance requires enough good sleep. In addition to promoting the synthesis of growth hormones and controlling cortisol levels, getting enough sleep also affects the balance of other hormones linked to metabolism, hunger control, and reproductive health. Hormonal balance may be upset by sleep disorders, which might affect general health.

Sleep Hygiene Practices

Hormonal balance and restful sleep are enhanced by implementing appropriate sleep hygiene habits, which include keeping a regular sleep schedule, establishing a calming bedtime ritual, and providing a pleasant sleeping environment. For better quality sleep, limit your time spent on devices and engage in stimulating activities before bedtime.

Weight Management and Hormonal Health

Hormonal imbalances in Obesity

Hormonal imbalances might result from being overweight. Hormones produced by adipose tissue may upset hormonal balance by promoting inflammation and altering insulin sensitivity. Hormonal equilibrium is supported by keeping a healthy body mass index (BMI) and controlling weight.

Metabolism and Hormones

Hormones are essential for controlling metabolism. Hormone imbalances such as those caused by insulin, leptin, or ghrelin may impact energy expenditure, appetite, and fat storage, ultimately impacting metabolic health and weight control. Lifestyle decisions that promote hormonal balance have a favorable effect on metabolism as well.

Environmental Factors and Hormonal Harmony

Toxins and Endocrine Disruptors

Hormone synthesis and signaling may be disrupted by exposure to environmental pollutants, such as endocrine-disrupting compounds found in certain plastics, insecticides, and personal care items. Reducing exposure to these drugs may help preserve hormonal balance.

Dietary Choices and Environmental Impact

Hormone balance may be preserved by limiting exposure to possible endocrine disruptors by selecting hormone-free goods, eating less pesticide-filled food, and sticking to an organic or minimally processed diet.

Hormonal equilibrium is crucial for overall health and well-being. Hormonal balance is greatly influenced by lifestyle choices, which have an impact on mood, energy levels, metabolism, and reproductive health, among other elements of health. A balanced diet, consistent exercise, efficient stress management, restful sleep, controlling weight, and reduced exposure to pollutants from the environment are all crucial for reaching and maintaining the ideal hormonal balance. People may support their general health and well-being and encourage hormonal equilibrium by implementing these lifestyle variables into their everyday routines. Hormonal balance must be achieved and maintained throughout life via a comprehensive approach to health that emphasizes these lifestyle variables.

Chapter 9

Lifelong Hormonal Health

An essential element of general well-being that is vital at every stage of life is hormonal health. Hormones are important messengers that coordinate a variety of physiological processes from early development through puberty, maturity, and old life. To ensure a balanced and healthy future, it is essential to comprehend the significance of preserving hormonal balance during all life stages. This thorough book explores the importance of hormonal health throughout life, explaining how hormones affect development, growth, mental stability, reproduction, and general health. We examine the elements that go into hormonal balance and provide guidance on how to build a future with ideal hormonal health.

Childhood Hormonal Health

Hormones have a crucial role in the growth and development of children. Growth and general height rise are fueled by growth hormone, which is produced by the pituitary gland. Thyroid hormones can have an impact on cognitive and physical development. But this period is not only about physical development; it's also when hormonal balance establishes the foundation for long-term health. It becomes crucial to guarantee that kids have access to nutritious, well-balanced food to support optimal hormonal development.

Adolescent Hormone Health

Hormonal volatility is particularly prominent during the childhood-adolescent transition. The hormones that lead to the development of secondary sexual traits, such as testosterone and estrogen, become more active. Hormonal changes can cause emotional and mood swings. This is a stage when complete knowledge of the shifting hormonal environment and education about reproductive health are crucial. Adolescents may make decisions that set the stage for a healthy hormonal future when they are equipped with correct knowledge of menstruation, sexual health, and contraception.

Health of the Hormones in Adulthood

Hormonal factors become more numerous when one reaches adulthood, especially when it comes to family planning. Estrogen, progesterone, and testosterone are reproductive hormones that become important decision-making factors. Understanding these hormones is essential for those who want to grow their families since they affect fertility and family size regulation. By controlling these hormones, hormonal contraceptive methods—such as birth control pills—provide family planning alternatives and increase reproductive control. Changes in hormones throughout pregnancy highlight how crucial it is to comprehend how these processes impact both the growing baby and the pregnant woman.

Middle-Aged Hormonal Health

Hormonal health poses distinct issues throughout middle age. Menopause in women is a normal process marked by a sharp drop in estrogen and progesterone levels. This drop in hormones may cause a variety of symptoms, such as mood swings and hot flashes. It's critical to control these hormonal fluctuations and how they affect general health. While it's not as well-defined as menopause, some men may go through andropause, which is a condition marked by a dip in testosterone levels. This hormone change may affect energy levels, muscular mass, and sexual health, among other areas of health. To properly manage men's health throughout middle age, it is important to comprehend these changes.

Hormonal Health in Older Age

Hormonal health also becomes important as one gets older. Hormonal changes have a major role in bone health. In women, a drop in estrogen and an increase in testosterone may lead to bone loss and an increased risk of osteoporosis. In later life, effective methods for preserving hormonal balance are essential. During this time, mood, general well-being, and cognitive performance may all be impacted by managing hormonal fluctuations. Lifestyle decisions that promote a balanced and healthy future may lessen the consequences of these hormone alterations. These decisions include eating a good diet, exercising often, engaging in cognitive stimulation, and limiting exposure to environmental contaminants.

Hormonal Balancing and Lifestyle Factors

Hormonal balance is greatly influenced by lifestyle choices throughout life. Hormonal health is greatly enhanced by a well-balanced diet high in vital nutrients, frequent exercise, efficient stress management, restful sleep, and avoiding environmental contaminants. These lifestyle decisions are essential to establishing and maintaining hormonal balance and a healthy future across all stages of life.

Hormone regulation affects development, maturation, mental health, sex, and general health throughout a lifetime. It's essential to comprehend how hormones function at every stage of life if you want to stay healthy. People may build a balanced and healthy future by making educated decisions, giving hormonal health priority, and getting medical help when necessary. To support hormonal balance throughout life, a comprehensive approach to health that includes nutrition, exercise, stress reduction, sleep, and avoiding environmental contaminants is essential. People may start a path toward a balanced and healthy future and embrace the many stages of life with elegance and vigor if they have a thorough awareness of the function hormones play in the body and the variables that affect them.

www.ingramcontent.com/pod-product-compliance
Lightning Source LLC
Chambersburg PA
CBHW070941260726
48661CB00003B/1070